Your ABC's to Happiness and Good Mental Health

T. L. FLOYD

PAGE PUBLISHING
Conneaut Lake, PA

First originally published by Page Publishing 2024

The content in this book should not be used as a replacement for professional medical or psychiatric advice, diagnosis or treatment. For medical advice, please consult a licensed healthcare specialist or a psychiatrist who specializes in mental health.

ISBN 979-8-89157-002-3 (pbk)
ISBN 979-8-89157-729-9 (hc)
ISBN 979-8-89157-014-6 (digital)

Printed in the United States of America

Dedication

To all the readers who pick up this book, always remember that the spirit of human beings thrives on hope, love, and kindness. Whenever help is needed, just open this book and be reminded that words have the power to change someone's heart, which will consequently change the world. It all begins with all of us!

Also available as an ebook, as an audiobook, professionally printed in hard copy and paperback editions, and as a compilation of voice-over narrator selection from Page Publishing, Inc.

Preface

We decided to write this book to help others since mental illness is on the rise in the United States and beyond. In this country, over 20 percent of people are experiencing some form of mental illness. In our opinion, the increase is due to the COVID-19 pandemic, latchkey children with little adult supervision, the rise in social media with inappropriate activity, smaller family units, and less community involvement due to societal trends.

Unfortunately, COVID-19 has devastated the world. It has changed the way we live our lives, how we communicate with others (example: Zoom), how our children are educated, how we care for others, how we perform at work and more. As a result, many people are suffering from mental health problems. For the above reasons, we were prompted to write this book. We want to provide information to help as many people as we can. If we can help one person with their happiness and good mental health, our mission will be accomplished!

The purpose for writing the *Your ABC's to Happiness and Good Mental Health* book is to boost your mood, handle your emotions better, build resilience, and help people get through tough times.

This book can help increase an individual's happiness, mental health, overall well-being, and satisfaction with life. It can help the reader manage difficult emotions when confronted with a new and rapidly changing reality. The content was written to make sure that its messages resonated with people of different age groups, different backgrounds, and continents.

As authors, we want to equip the readers with life-changing strategies to help show how to enhance their mood and their ability to cope with stress. The book can help them overcome challenges, build relationships, and recover from life's setbacks and hardships.

Being happy and mentally healthy don't require winning the lottery or some other drastic change of circumstances. What it takes is an inner change of your attitude and perspective. This is good news, because it's something all of us can do.

Remember: If you're having a bad day, you are the only one who can fix it and make it better.

Daily Habits

The following daily habits may help you achieve more happiness and good mental health in your life one day at a time. It can be as easy as learning your ABC's.

_A_ is for _acknowledgment_ and _avoid_. It is important to acknowledge the unhappy moments and allow yourself to experience it for a short period of time. Then shift your focus toward what made you feel this way in the first place and what it might take to recover. For an example, would a deep breathing exercise help? Can you talk it over with someone you can trust? Can you make time for a long walk outside? Or will reading _Your ABC's to Happiness and Good Mental Health_ book help out?

Let the moment pass and take care of yourself. Remember, no one's happy all the time.

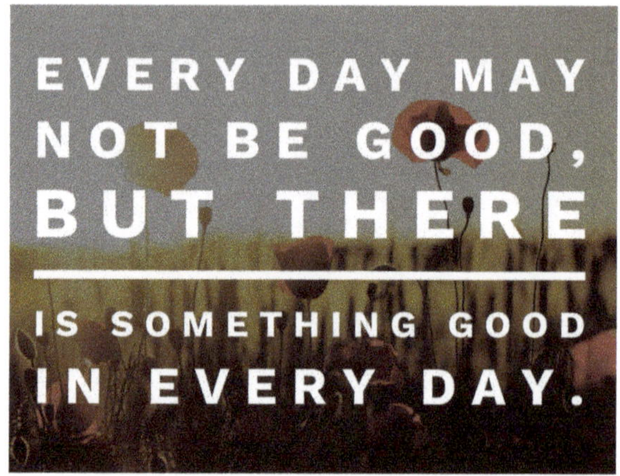

Quote - "Every day may not be good, but there is something good in every day." Meaningful quote for life learning.

**Avoid**. Avoid comparing yourself to others. When you acknowledge your unhappy moment and deal with it in a timely fashion, it is beneficial for your inner peace and happiness.

_B_ is for _breathing_. Slow breathing and breathing deep exercises can help reduce stress. Also, breathing exercises allow you to reduce feelings of anxiety and to think more clearly.

Controlled breathing can be used to improve vitality and promote concentration. Breathing practices can help reduce symptoms associated with anxiety, insomnia, post-traumatic stress disorder, depression, and attention-deficit disorder.

It has been proven that our brain associates different emotions with different breathing patterns, and breathing exercises work because they trick your brain into thinking your emotional state is different than it actually is at the current time. When we are happy, our breathing is steady and regular. However, when we are fearful, stressed and anxious, our breathing becomes quicker, irregular, and shallow. You can trick your brain into thinking you're actually in a calm state and there is no threat or challenge at hand when you slow your breathing down in times of stressful situations.

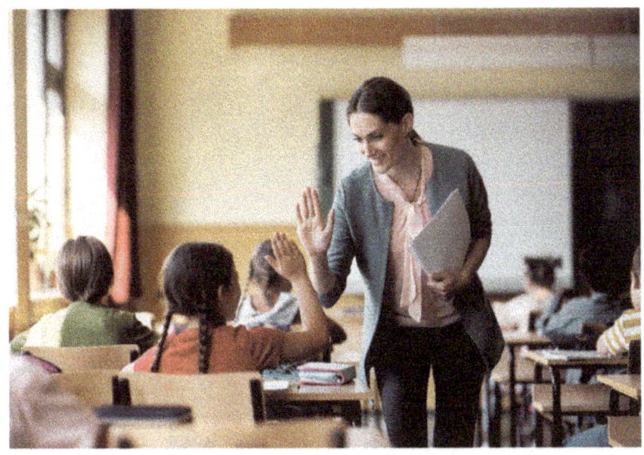

Picture of a happy elementary school teacher giving high-five to her student during class in the classroom.

_C_ is for _compliment_ and _confidence_. Giving a sincere compliment is a quick, easy way to brighten someone's day while giving your own happiness a boost. Compliments feel good because they activate reward areas in the brain, such as the striatum. However, giving people compliments not only makes them feel good, it also helps them to learn and acquire new skills. And as if that weren't enough, you can also use compliments to improve the ambiance or to reinforce desired behavior in others.

Sometimes all it takes to brighten up our day is a kind word, a sincere praise, a grateful smile. We have all seen time and again that the simple act of appreciating someone's effort can have a huge transformative effect on their attitude and productivity.

Compliments are powerful. They have the ability to change the very fabric of our brains in ways that are not always apparent but go a long way. They not only make us feel good, but also significantly impact memory, learning, motivation, and other cognitive functions. We should compliment people often, which helps enhance happiness and good mental health.

Let's open our eyes and hearts. We should find the good in people around us and appreciate them for who they are, and not be judgmental. A little appreciation goes a long way in making people feel and act better. So let's praise away for a better, healthier, and happier world!

Confidence. The relationship between happiness and confidence is very important. Studies confirm that higher self-confidence and self-esteem predict a higher level of happiness. Self-confidence is hugely important to having a happy and successful life and career. Self-confidence exists whether you are aware of your own or not. Increase your self-confidence and you can increase the quality of your life.

Confident individuals tend to be more emotionally stable, have a more constructive outlook, and feel greater self-acceptance and respect. Because of the above, they are also able to focus on the positives in life, to enjoy greater relationships, to compare themselves less to the Joneses, and to seek enrichment through experiences and self-improvement. They are simply better equipped to deal with life, manage stress, and reach their goals.

All these benefits that confidence brings translate into improved long-term well-being and life satisfaction. We can live a good life which gives us a sense of joy, peace with ourselves, excitement, and gratitude. In other words, confidence leads us to happiness and good mental health.

_D_ is for _decision-making skills_ and _declutter_. Since life is full of choices, it is important to know how to make good decisions. Some decisions are easier than others, such as what outfit to wear or what to have for dinner. Other decisions are more difficult, like which college to attend, choosing a career, or who to marry. Regardless of how important a decision is, having good decision-making skills are extremely useful in life situations.

Decluttering is a process of keeping what you really love and then creating a way to store it. It sounds like a big project, but setting aside just twenty minutes a week can have a big impact. When you have less stuff, you have more clarity because you're not thinking about all your stuff.

People can feel so overwhelmed by their stuff. When they start to declutter, the initial feeling is hope that their life will be changed by doing the work. They also begin to feel a greater sense of control and well-being by lowering their stress levels. After all, there's nothing more stressful than searching for your keys as you're trying to get out of the house on time.

E is for *education*, *exercise*, and *eat*. Educate yourself by learning something new every day. As you age, learning something new every day is a great way to keep your brain sharp. If you practice this on a regular basis, you can improve your memory, concentration, and problem solving. Also, this practice may reduce the chance of developing dementia. Your brain will be preserved for years to come if you keep it engaged.

Exercise. Exercise isn't just for your body; regular exercise can help reduce stress, feelings of anxiety, and symptoms of depression while boosting self-esteem and happiness. It's not certain if moving makes you happy or if happy people just move more, but it is known that more activity goes hand in hand with better health and greater happiness.

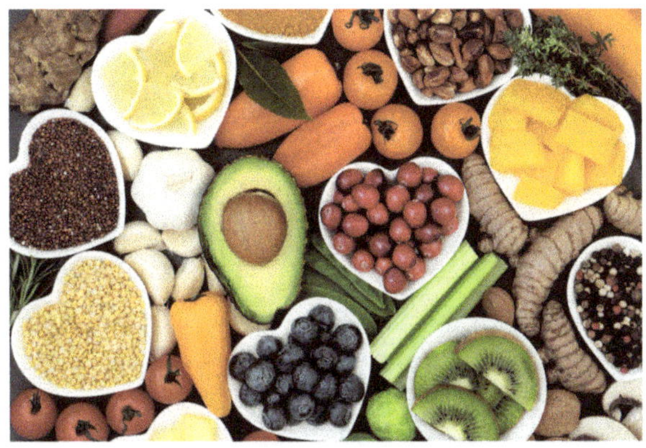

Picture of healthy food for fitness concept with immune boosting properties with fruit, vegetables, herbs, spice, and grains.

Eat. Eat with mood in mind. Eat a diet that is rich in brain food such as fish, seafood, beans, legumes, leafy greens, and other vegetables, olive oil (monounsaturated fat), yogurt, and nuts. These foods can be an effective and relatively simple way to promote mental health and recovery from mental illness that can easily be integrated into your health care.

F is for ***face stress head-on***, ***focus***, and ***fun***. It is important to face stress head-on. This might mean initiating an uncomfortable conversation or putting in some extra work, but the sooner you confront it, the sooner the pit in your stomach may start to shrink.

Focus. Focus on the good. There are good things in your life right now: you are alive, you are fed, you are healthy, you have family and friends, and you have opportunities each day to pursue meaningful work. Maybe not all those are true for you right now, but some of them are a part of your life. This means there is good in your life that you can focus on right now.

There was a man who came home from the war. He said that people would ask him, "How can you stay so positive after losing your legs?" He responded by asking them how they can stay so negative when they have both of their legs. He did a great job putting it all into perspective.

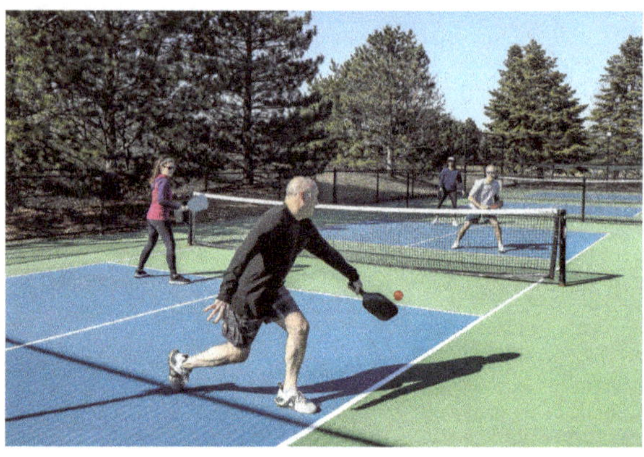

Picture of a player hitting a backhand in a competitive doubles game of pickleball with a group of men and women on a blue and green court.

Fun! Laughing with friends, throwing a ball for the dog, watching your favorite TV show, playing softball, pickleball, or reading a book might be called leisure activities, but the health benefits associated with some good old-fashioned fun are nothing short of incredible.

Having fun increases serotonin levels. Serotonin is a chemical that regulates many of our most basic processes—including sleep patterns, memory, body temperature, and mood. Doing activities that you enjoy will help you relax and connect with others. This will naturally increase the body's serotonin levels.

- Laughing decreases pain, may help your heart and lungs, promotes muscle relaxation, and can reduce anxiety.
- Positive emotions can decrease stress hormones and build emotional strength.
- Leisure activities offer a distraction from problems, a sense of competence, and many other benefits. For example, one twin who participated in leisure activities and eat healthy may be less likely to develop Alzheimer's disease or other health illnesses than his twin who lives far away and practices an unhealthy lifestyle.

Just like healthy eating is most beneficial when done over a sustained period of time, the health benefits of having fun only improve with time. Making a habit of relaxing, engaging in activities you enjoy, and spending time with people who make you happy will yield sustained and increasingly positive benefits of consistently lower stress, positive feelings, better sleep, better coping abilities, and improved relationships.

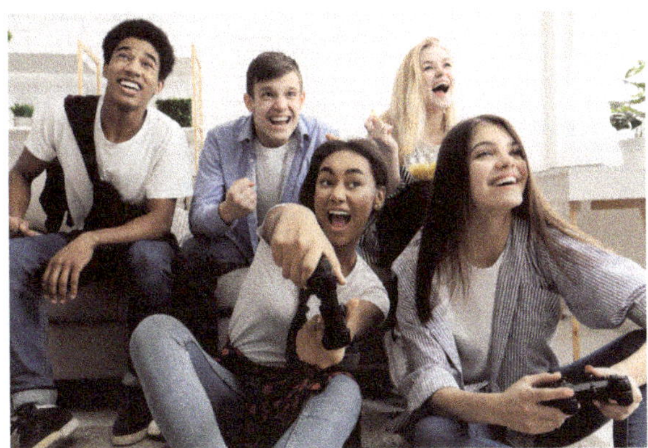

Picture of playful teenage friends playing online
video games and having fun at home.

Having fun and experiencing good times build relationships, and good relationships are key to our happiness and good mental health.

_G_ is for being _grateful_ and _giving back to society_. Practicing gratitude is meaningful. Simply being grateful can give your mood a big boost. It can have a significant impact on feelings of hope and happiness. Be grateful for what you have, appreciate who you are, work hard every day to live your best life, and stop comparing yourself to others. Gratitude and generosity can only be understood correctly when we see them as disciplines rather than responses. A discipline is something we practice regardless of our circumstances. If you are waiting for enough money to become generous, you'll never get there. Likewise, if you are waiting for everything to be perfect to be grateful, you'll never experience it. Choose to be thankful today. And choose to be generous with your time and money. Making them both a discipline in your life will result in a happier today and tomorrow.

Give back to society. True meaning in life doesn't come from what you get; it comes from what you give. The importance of giving back to society enables you to better the lives of the people around you. You can help the people you love, the ones in your community, or anywhere else in the world. Giving back doesn't just benefit others, it also helps you.

H **is for *happiness* and *healthy*.** Happiness is a state of mind. Happiness is a choice. Specifically, it is a state of contentment and well-being. Happy people focus on positive thoughts. Happiness starts with a healthy lifestyle. Doing things that you enjoy is good for your emotional well-being. Simple activities like watching sports with a friend, taking a relaxing bubble bath, or meeting up with friends for coffee can all improve your day.

Doing something you're good at, such as cooking, singing, playing sports, or dancing is a good way to enjoy yourself and have a sense of achievement.

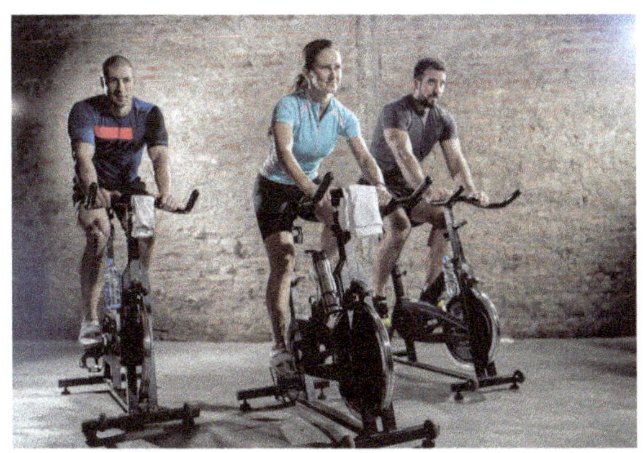

Picture of young people cycling workout with rhythm of powerful music.

Healthy. Getting sweaty feels good. It really does! Being physically active causes chemical changes in the brain which can help improve your mood. It also brings a sense of greater self-esteem. There is a strong relationship between physical activity and mental wellness. Being more physically active improves heart health, blood pressure, and some joint-related pain. It also enhances blood sugar control and weight loss.

Get plenty of sleep; most people need at least seven hours of sleep every night. Adequate sleep is vital to good health, brain function, and emotional well-being. Getting enough sleep also reduces your risk of developing certain chronic illnesses, such as heart disease, depression, and diabetes.

Try some of the following suggestions: Spend time outside, eat healthy meals, exercise regularly, put down your cell phone, work hard, play harder, have fun, pray often, and rest your body. When you make the suggestions a part of your lifestyle, you'll be surprised how your happiness, well-being, and good mental health levels will be enhanced.

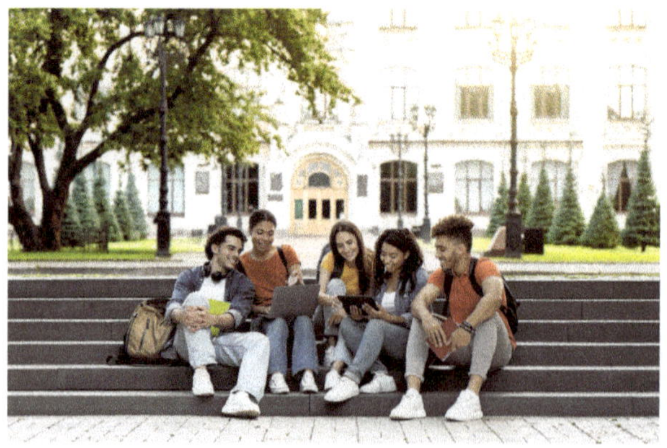

Picture of college students using Digital Tablet and Laptop studying together outdoors. Happy friends sitting on stairs near university building using modern gadgets for education.

I is for ***intelligence*** and ***integrity***. People who are intelligent and exhibit higher IQ tend to be more successful in life. Success in life contributes to happiness. It is safe to conclude that high IQ is associated with factors that contribute to happiness, success, and good mental health.

Integrity. Integrity is a core quality required for a happy and successful life. It is the single most valuable character a person can develop to remarkably enhance all parts of their lives. When you decide to be a person of integrity and then commit to it, you will have taken the first step to a much more successful life.

When you live a life of integrity, you're truthful and clear about who you are or your stance on a matter. Your day-to-day life becomes easier, and you are at peace because you do not have to worry about hiding anything.

Excellent relationships develop when you live a life of integrity. We are often attracted to people who have good morals and values like us. Living in integrity shows commendable character, and you will naturally draw people to you. When you do not have to compromise on your values to have friends or be dishonest, you'll find out that you'll have high-quality and better relationships.

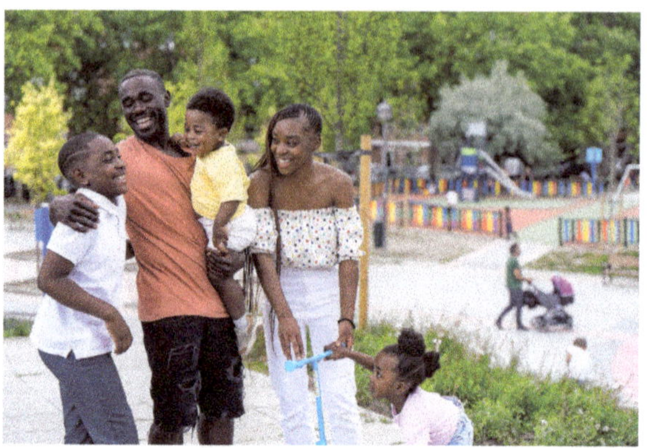

Picture of a family of five having fun with happy children together at the playground.

J **is for** *joy* **and** *journaling*. Joy is an emotional response that typically arises when something positive has happened to you or to someone important to you. It also arises when your needs are met. Thus, the feeling of joy makes you seek more of it and to know what's important to you.

Someone who's joyful is very happy. A joyful child will laugh with delight. For many people, their wedding day, the birth of their children, doing well on an exam, a lovely sunset, or simply a beautiful summer afternoon can all be joyful occasions.

Joyful people are often loving people because they are able to appreciate others despite their flaws and transgressions. They are able to look past the negative aspects of a person or situation and find the good. Joyful people do not judge others, but they are kind, generous, caring, and compassionate towards everyone.

Journaling*.* A journal is a good way to organize your thoughts, analyze your feelings, and make plans.

Plan ahead and write down the things that you will be doing tomorrow. Get a good night's sleep, wake up, eat a healthy breakfast, be grateful, think positive thoughts, avoid negativity, listen to your favorite song, and exercise.

Also, it can be as simple as jotting down a few thoughts before you go to bed. If putting certain things in writing makes you nervous, you can always shred it when you've finished. It's the process that counts. When you start adopting these little things into your day, you can begin to live a joyful and a happier life!

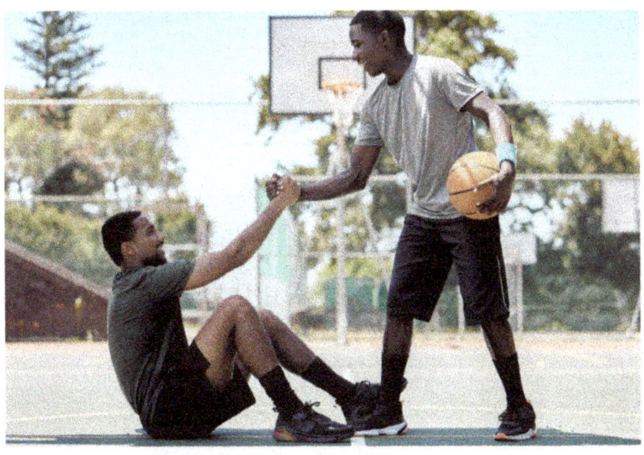

Picture of two happy friends playing basketball on the outdoor basketball court. They exhibit teamwork, helping hand, support, respect, trust, kindness, and assistance in competition training games.

_K_ is for _kindness_. Performing acts of kindness can help promote your overall well-being. You can forget many things in life, but you will never forget kindness.

Even the smallest acts of kindness can make you feel happy and improve your mental health. It could be as simple as a friendly smile or holding the door for another person. Demonstrating acts of kindness truly brings happiness and good mental health to those who practice it on a regular basis.

Kindness has been shown to increase empathy, self-esteem, and compassion and improve your mood. It can decrease cortisol. Cortisol is a stress hormone which directly impacts stress levels.

Doing nice things for others boosts your serotonin. Serotonin is the neurotransmitter responsible for feelings of satisfaction and well-being. Also, people who give of themselves in a balanced way tend to be healthier and happier, exhibit good mental health, and they live longer.

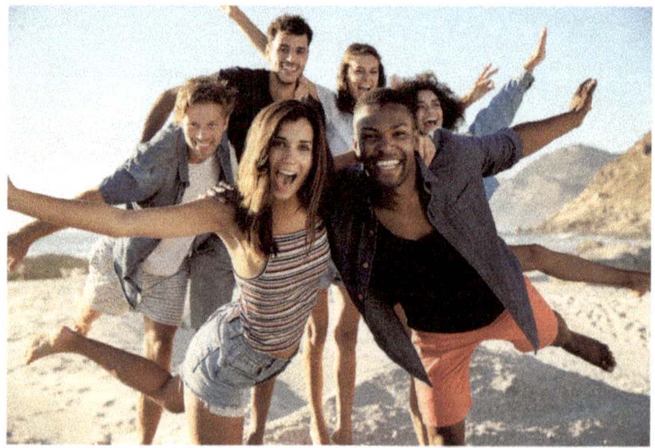

Picture of friends having fun together on a beach vacation with arms outstretched.

_L_ is for _laughter_ and _learning new things_. Laughing sends more oxygen to the brain, and that triggers the release of endorphins, or brain chemicals that help us feel positive. Laughing can also lower blood pressure, relieve stress, temporarily relieve pain, and boost mood.

People with a strong sense of humor outlived those who don't laugh as much. Laughter improves the function of blood vessels and increases blood flow, which can help protect you against a heart attack and other cardiovascular problems.

Nothing diffuses anger and conflict faster than a shared laugh. Looking at the funny side can put problems into perspective and enable you to move on from confrontations without holding on to bitterness or resentment.

Laughter stops distressing emotions. You can't feel anxious, angry, or sad when you're laughing. Laughter helps you relax and recharge. It reduces stress and increases energy, enabling you to stay focused and accomplish more.

Laughter shifts perspective, allowing you to see situations in a more realistic, less threatening light. A humorous perspective creates psychological distance, which can help you avoid feeling overwhelmed and diffuse conflict.

Laughter makes you feel happy, and it draws you closer to others, which can have a profound effect on all aspects of your mental and emotional health.

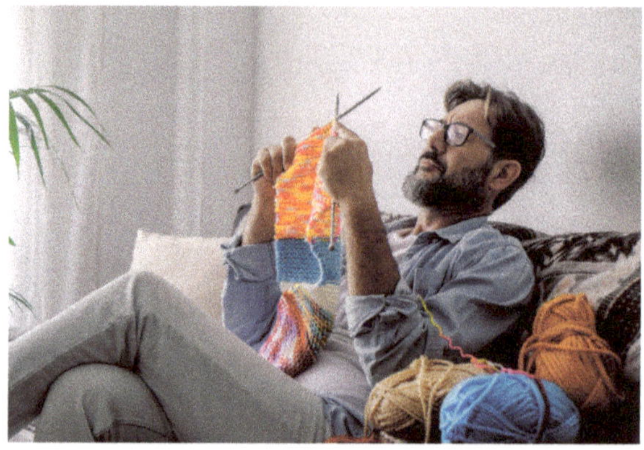

Picture of a man sitting and relaxing on the sofa learning a new skill. He is learning how to knit with colorful wool.

Learning new things. Living a happier and more satisfied life can start with learning new things. Engaging in mentally stimulating activities, such as reading, learning to play a musical instrument, playing brain or board games, or even socializing with people can all create new brain connections. So whether you learn a new language, take up a new sport, or volunteer for a project that involves a skill you don't usually use, you're building cognitive reserve, which is associated with lower rates of dementia and better thinking skills. Don't forget to experiment with things that require manual dexterity as well as mental effort, such as painting, drawing, knitting, and other crafts.

Having a job keeps you mentally active, but it's wise to get in the habit of trying new things so that when you retire, you're likely to keep learning.

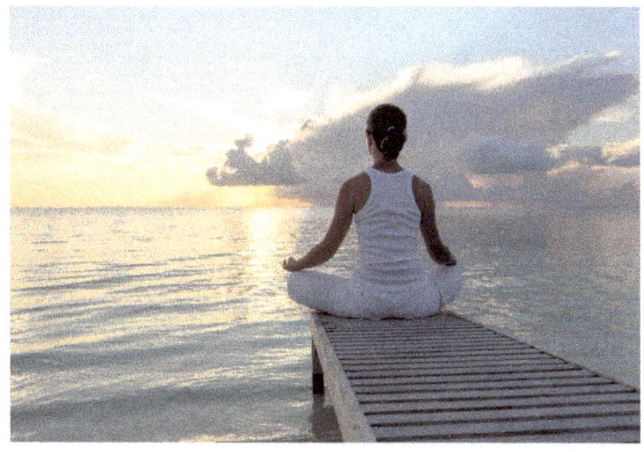

Picture of a woman meditating while practicing yoga at the seashore.

_M_ is for _meditation_ and _memory_. Meditation doesn't have to be complicated. It can be as simple as sitting quietly with your own thoughts for five minutes. Even the deep breathing exercises mentioned earlier can serve as a form of meditation.

Memory. Happy memories are essential to our good mental health. When we savor our positive memories, we can increase positive emotions. For example, you begin to smile while looking through your high school or college yearbook or your wedding photo album or seeing pictures of your children, family members, and friends. These photos tend to provide opportunities for you to reminisce on the fun times that were had, thus making you smile, feel good, and be happy.

Good memories have the capacity to reduce anxiety by reducing the way we attend to and experience threat. It can ease the symptoms of depression by letting the world be seen through a more positive filter.

A good working memory could be the secret to a more successful and joyful life. People with a good working memory are more likely to be self-assured, optimistic, and happier.

N **is for** *nature*. Get into nature. Spending thirty minutes or more a week in green spaces can help lower blood pressure and the chances of developing depression.

O **is for** *optimistic*, *open minded*, **and** *organized*. Optimism and the ability to learn how to tame negative thoughts should be approached every day. Happiness often comes from within.

Thinking positive thoughts and surrounding yourself with positive people really does help. Optimism, like pessimism, can be infectious, so make a point to hang out with optimistic people.

Open minded. An open mind is a pathway to possibility. Be open to new people, places, and experiences. When you are flexible and open to change, your happiness can increase.

Organized. Being organized can benefit your health and help you feel happier and more relaxed. Get in the habit of writing things down. You will be amazed at how much more you remember and how organized your life becomes.

You can start organizing and freshening up your life today. Start evaluating where you can improve and begin to make small yet impactful changes to have a more organized lifestyle. This will help alleviate stress and improve your mood, happiness, and mental health.

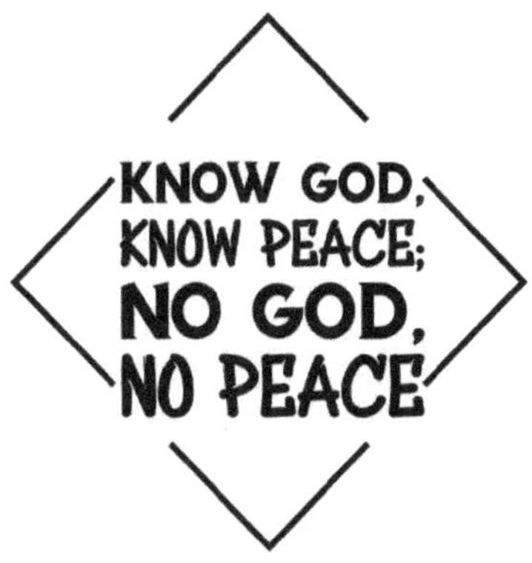

Quote - "Know God, Know Peace; No God; No Peace."

_P_ is for _power of prayer_, _positivity_, and _politeness_. The power of prayer can make you happier, calmer, and better equipped to deal with the problems life presents. When prayer elicits feelings of love and compassion, there is a release of serotonin and dopamine. Both of these neurotransmitters play a role in how you feel. Serotonin has a direct impact on your mood, and not having enough serotonin has been linked to depression. Dopamine, on the other hand, is associated with reward and motivation.

Prayer can also boost overall happiness, especially when we define happiness as having meaning and connection in one's life. Living a life of meaning and purpose contributes to overall positive feelings, and praying to a higher power is based on the belief that there is something greater than one's everyday life and stressors. When praying, a person focuses on the bigger picture of what is important, which counters the taxing minutiae of everyday life.

Prayer can influence numerous areas of our lives, all of which contribute to our overall positive emotions. It can help someone feel connected to a source of unconditional love, reduce emotional distress, serve as a healthy coping mechanism, enhance one's sense of self, boost one's happiness in relationships, and encourage positive behaviors.

Positivity. Positive people are more hopeful, have more energy, and are more self-confident. Because of this, they tend to set higher goals and spend more effort in order to reach their goals. Also, they are more resilient, which helps them bounce back and persevere despite setbacks.

Positive thinking is important because it can have a beneficial impact on both physical and mental well-being. People who maintain a more positive outlook on life cope better with stress, have better immunity, and have a lower risk of premature death.

A positive attitude helps to cope with the daily affairs of life. It brings optimism into your life and makes it easier to avoid worry and negative thinking. Adopting positive thoughts for your way of living will bring constructive changes into your days and make you happier, successful, and it enhances good mental health.

Politeness. The lack of politeness today is shocking. For example, road rage incidents have increased recently. This proves that society has forgotten how to be nice.

It doesn't take much effort to be polite. In fact, it's something that we teach children. When you think about it, being polite simply means interacting positively with others. Saying thank you with a smile is the least you can do.

Look for ways to be polite and lend a helping hand. It can be something as simple as helping someone pick up a dropped item or holding the door for someone. Make it about them and not yourself.

_Q_ is for _quality of life_ and _quiet time_. People with a higher quality of life or well-being mostly claim to be content with their lives. Also, they are happier and more productive at work or at school.

Quiet time. Quiet time allows you to be alone with your thoughts and take a break from your frazzled routine. You may feel more creative, less tense, and have better focus and attention. Actively choosing silence over noise can be empowering, calming, and revitalizing.

Quiet time is healthy for body and mind. Silence offers opportunities for self-reflection and daydreaming, which activates multiple parts of the brain. It gives us time to turn down the inner noise and increase awareness of what matters most.

_R_ is for _respect_ and _relationships_. Respect can be defined as thinking and feeling good things about a person. Also, it's treating someone in a way that shows them that you care about their well-being. When you respect someone, you consider them as a person of worth. Respect creates a positive environment in which relationships can flourish. Without it, relationships can struggle.

Before you can respect others, you have to respect yourself. You can't think positively about others if you don't think positively about yourself. Basically, a person that respects themselves will treat others the way they want to be treated.

In short, self-respect means having confidence and behaving with dignity. When you respect yourself, you believe that you're worthy of being respected and loved. Without it, you won't be able to accept the respect that others have for you. In turn, you won't respect others because you won't understand the positive effects that respect has on a person.

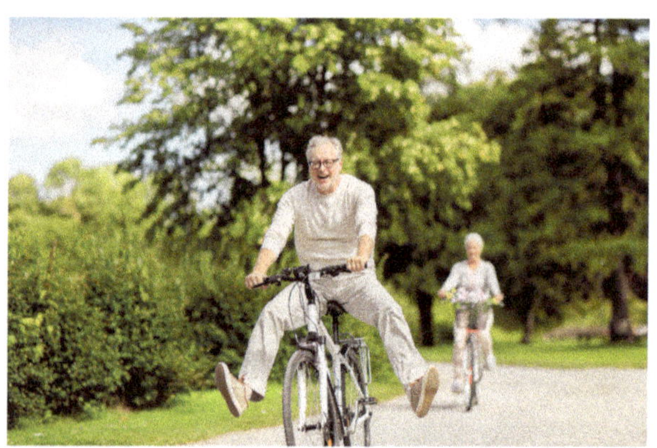

Picture of active and happy senior couple riding bicycles at summer park.

Relationships. Relationships hold the key to happiness, and recognizing the best in everyone leads to healthier relationships. Close relationships, more than money or fame, are what keep people happy throughout their lives. Those ties protect people from life's discontents, help to delay mental and physical decline, and are better predictors of long and happy lives than social class, IQ, or even genes.

Humans are largely considered social beings. Social relationships can make us happy. Take time to visit with family members and friends.

Companionship doesn't have to be limited to other humans. Pets can offer similar benefits. More information in reference to the benefits of pets is mentioned in the letter *Z* below.

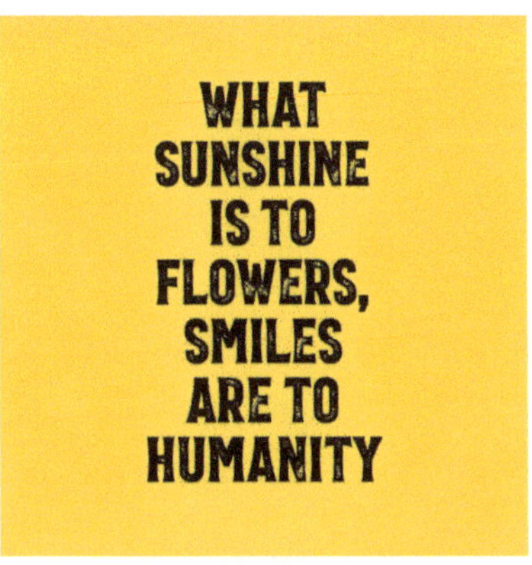

Quote - "What sunshine is to flowers, smiles are to humanity."

_S_ is for _smile_ and _self-care_. We smile because we're happy, and smiling causes the brain to release dopamine, which makes us happier.

Smiling makes us feel really good. It has health benefits, inflicts happiness on those around us, and makes us look younger! We were born to smile. In fact, we actually smile in the womb and in our sleep as a young baby. So it is life that teaches us not to smile, and with this in mind, we can also train ourselves to smile more! This is a satisfying truth.

According to the well-known smile expert, it is stated that the act of smiling itself actually makes us feel better rather than smiling being merely a result of feeling good. Smiling releases endorphins, natural painkillers, and serotonin, three neurotransmitters that make us feel good from head to toe. These natural chemicals elevate our mood, relax our body, and reduce physical pain. Consider smiling as a natural drug. One single smile is as stimulating to our brain as eating chocolate candy bars or winning thousands of dollars. Wow!

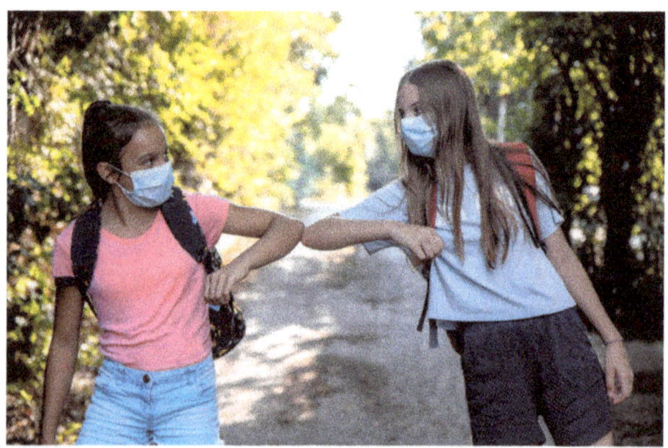

Picture of two teenage girls touching elbows and wearing masks. The touching of the elbows is a new safety protective behavior due to the Covid-19 pandemic.

___**Self-care**___. It's easy to neglect self-care in a fast-paced world. But trying to find time to nurture yourself as much as you can is important in supporting your body's responsibilities of carrying your thoughts, passions, and spirit through this world.

T **is for *therapy*.** You don't need to have a diagnosed mental health condition or overwhelming crisis to seek therapy. There is a stigma attached to mental illness which prevents those who need the services to reach out for help. They are too concerned about what others may think of them. It is important to seek mental help because the mental health professionals are trained to help people improve coping skills. Plus, there's no obligation to continue once you start. Even just a few sessions can help you add some new goodies to your emotional toolbox.

U **is for *universe* and *unconditional love*.** The size of our universe (and happiness) begins to expand when we serve others without concern over what we might receive in return; we experience the beauty of selfless love.

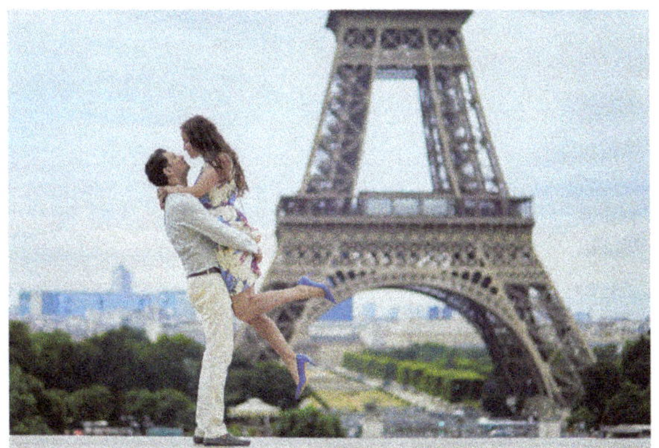

Picture of a happy romantic couple expressing love by hugging near the Eiffel tower in Paris.

Unconditional love. Unconditional love is important because it affects so many aspects of happiness and good mental and physical health. Evidence shows that unconditional love is one of the most powerful factors in healthy development for children and teens. Children who receive unconditional love from their parents have better stress resilience, better health, stronger self-esteem, stronger immune system, and better brain development.

_V_ is for *volunteering*. Volunteering is another way to connect with others. Just as we're hardwired to be social, we're also hardwired to give to others. The meaning and purpose derived from helping others or the community can enrich and expand your life. Volunteering makes you happier. There's no limit to the individual and group volunteer opportunities you can explore. Schools, churches, nonprofits, and charitable organizations of all sorts depend on volunteers for their survival.

Giving to others can also help protect your mental, physical, and social health. It can reduce stress, combat depression, keep you mentally stimulated, increase the opportunity to meet new people, and provide a sense of purpose. While it's true that the more you volunteer, the more benefits you'll experience, volunteering doesn't have to involve a long-term commitment or take a huge amount of time out of your busy day. Giving in simple ways can help those in need and improve your health and happiness.

Volunteering makes you happy. By measuring hormones and brain activity, researchers have discovered that being helpful to others delivers immense pleasure. Human beings are hardwired to give to others. The more we give, the happier we feel.

_W_ is for _weekly planning, worry less, winner, and water_. Try sitting down at the end of every week and making a basic list for the following week. Even if you don't stick to the plan, blocking out time where you can do laundry, go grocery shopping, study for a test, or tackle projects at work or school can help quiet your mind.

Worry less. Worry about nothing. Constant worrying, negative thinking, and always expecting the worst can take a toll on your emotional and physical health. It can sap your emotional strength, leave you feeling restless and jumpy, cause insomnia, headaches, stomach problems, and muscle tension, and make it difficult to concentrate at work or school.

Stop worrying about the future because you cannot control the future. Luck, randomness, and chance contribute so much to the unpredictable nature of life that it is just unrealistic to think you can control things.

Ultimately, the goal is to let go of a chronic negative mindset and learn how to cultivate and savor more positive emotional states. This may mean facing your fears. This will allow you to relax and let your guard down and to let yourself feel emotionally vulnerable. (Remember, it sometimes takes courage to be happy.)

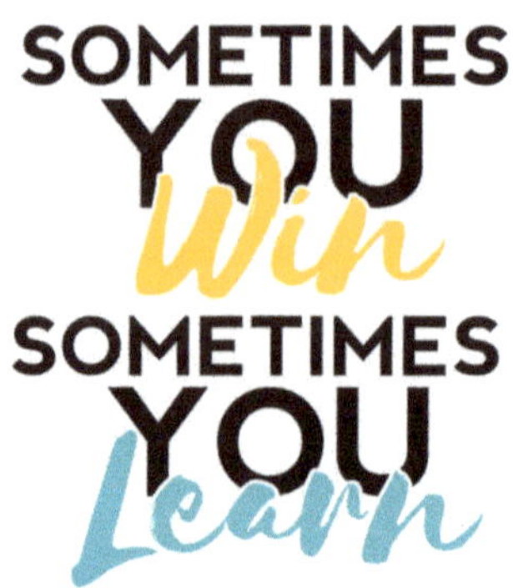

Quote - "Sometimes you win, sometimes you learn."

Winner. To win the race, you must have a winner's mindset. You must be able to see yourself at the finish line. You must determine in your mind that nothing will get in your way to slow you down. If at first you don't succeed, you must pick yourself up, dust yourself off, and try again. You know who you are, believe in yourself, and persevere to the end. Finishing strong takes this victorious winner's mindset.

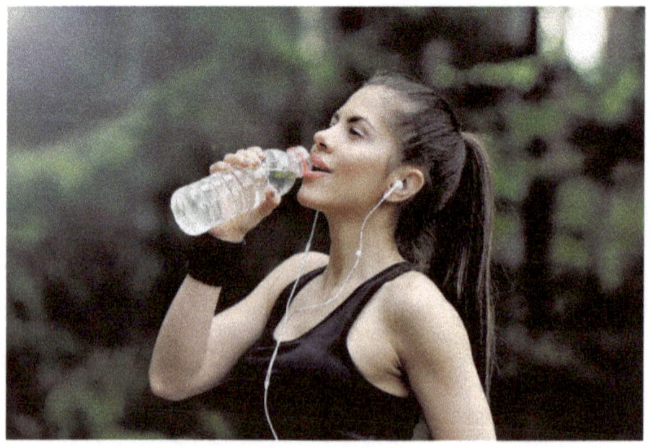

Picture of a fitness sporty woman running in a forest area drinking water.

Water. Drinking water stimulates the flow of nutrients and hormones that generate endorphins in your brain and leave you feeling happy. It helps you stay awake, boosts your daily productivity, and flushes out harmful toxins.

Time spent near water is the secret of happiness. Spending time in and around aquatic environments has consistently been shown to lead to significantly higher benefits, inducing positive mood and reducing negative mood and stress better than green space does. People of all socioeconomic groups go to the coast to spend quality time with friends and family.

Whether it's a bathtub, a pool, or an ocean, water makes us calmer. It makes us happier. It enhances our relationships. Research has shown that being near, in, on, or under water can lower stress, increase our sense of well-being and boost creativity.

Water has been shown to have natural calming properties. Drinking enough water is an important step in managing your anxiety. Even if you're not experiencing anxiety, drinking sufficient water can create feelings of relaxation.

People living near water have a lower risk of premature death, a lower risk of obesity, and generally report better mental health and well-being.

Studies have shown that dehydration leads to higher cortisol levels, the stress hormone, making it harder to deal with everyday issues. By staying hydrated, you will be better equipped to deal with everyday problems.

_**X**_ **is for _x-factor_**. X-factor is the thing that makes an individual stand out. The power to achieve everyday success and happiness is an x-factor that everyone can strive to achieve.

_**Y**_ **is for _your phone should be ditched_**. Really, unplug it. If you haven't unplugged in a while, you might be surprised at the difference it makes. Let your mind wander free for a change. Read a book, meditate, take a walk while paying attention to your surroundings. Spend time with and communicate with a friend in person—no texting allowed. Also, you can choose to be alone to meditate on ways to become a better you.

_**Z**_ **is for _zestful_ and _zoo_**. A zestful person has enthusiasm and energy. They are likely to wake up feeling active and willing to take on the day. They will work with high spirits and have the solidarity to confront difficulty. Zest is an essential component of positive psychology and a standout among our most instrumental character qualities.

A zest for living and the ability to laugh and have fun are very important. The joyful energy of zest is good for happiness and for good mental health!

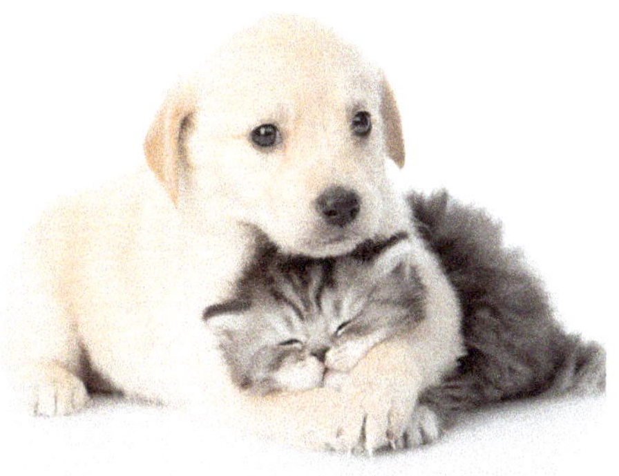

A super cute picture of a golden retriever puppy hugging a British cat!

Zoo. Zoo visits can help improve a person's overall well-being. It is no secret that animals can help people with their happiness, mental, physical, social, and emotional health. Studies show that dogs are known to reduce anxiety, stress, and depression in people. Also, they can encourage exercise, ease loneliness, and improve your health overall. For example, dog owners are less likely to develop heart disease, and they tend to have lower blood pressure.

So take some time from your business schedule and visit the zoo or adopt an animal from the animal shelter or rescue. It is a win-win situation. It will benefit you in many ways. As mentioned earlier, not only do animals give you unconditional love, but they have been shown to be psychologically, emotionally, and physically, and socially beneficial to their companions. Caring for a pet can provide a sense of purpose and fulfillment and lessen feelings of loneliness. And when you adopt, you can also feel proud about helping an animal in need!

The animal will be happy to be a part of a family that provides unconditional love and acceptance to their pet and welcome them into their forever homes!

Conclusion

After reading this book, it is our hope that you will take away some reasons why maintaining good mental health is important. It can help you perform daily tasks with ease, and it can help you cope with the stresses of life.

Keep in mind that your happiness is a personal decision. You can decide whether or not you want to be happy. Take care of your physical, mental, social, and emotional health. Stay in good relationships by surrounding yourself with kind and caring people. Maintaining positive mental health helps establish continued well-being and independence. Stay involved and make meaningful contributions to your community. Realize what you can do as a person. Take care of yourself and work in a productive manner to help others along the way.

About the Author

T. Floyd, MEd, is a mother of two amazing young men and two beautiful grandchildren. She has been married to her husband for thirty-six years. She attended college on full volleyball, softball, and academic scholarships. Presently, she is still an active softball player and loves the camaraderie that exists between her teammates. She is a retired educator from the Palm Beach County School District. She has thirty-six years of teaching experience in the state of Florida.

L. Floyd wrote his first poem when he was in elementary school titled "Why Did the Twin Towers Have to Fall?" It was acknowledged by President George W. Bush. As he grew older, he developed a strong passion for the game of football, which rewarded him with several athletic scholarships to play the game that he loves. He played in two college national championship games and was the victor of one. He married his college sweetheart, and they went on to have two beautiful children. Today, he puts his family first and writes different books and poetry. He resides in the beautiful Colorado Springs, Colorado.

Over the years, T. Floyd has taught her students the importance of being happy and learning more strategies to stay positive, which will improve their good mental health.

Through football, L. Floyd gave back to his community by motivating kids to perform well in school, graduate, and go on to attend college. He encouraged them to believe in themselves and to live a successful and healthy lifestyle. He gained a true sense of accomplishment that came from knowing that he made a difference in the lives of the children he mentored. This mother-and-son duo (T. and L. Floyd) collaborated on their life-experience efforts to produce this book. They were inspired to write the *Your ABCs to Happiness and Good Mental Health* book to continue her legacy by providing a resource that can be used to help others navigate more easily through the complexities of life.